Plant Based Diet for Beginners

Discover the Basics & Easiest Recipes to Start a New Life

By

Spoons of happiness

of inattention or otherwise, by any usage or abuse of any policies, processes, or directions contained within is the solitary and utter responsibility of the recipient reader. Under no circumstances will any legal responsibility or blame be held against the publisher for any reparation, damages, or monetary loss due to the information herein, either directly or indirectly.

Respective authors own all copyrights not held by the publisher.

The information herein is offered for informational purposes solely and is universal as so. The presentation of the information is without contract or any type of guarantee assurance.

The trademarks that are used are without any consent and the publication of the trademark is without permission or backing by the trademark owner. All trademarks and brands within this book are for clarifying purposes only and are owned by the owners themselves, not affiliated with this document.

Table of Contents

Introduction

Did you ever feel without enough energy for your daily routine?

Do you think that fast and processed food is the only thing that can fit your busy lifestyle?

Have you ever felt like none of the fad meal plans look like you?

Well, you have found the hidden treasure. This book will show you the nutritional content of all preparations and you will be able to buy how fast food and highly processed foods generate various health problems that probably affect the majority in your environment.

Increase your vital energy by changing your diet to a Plant Based Diet, which is not only a way of eating, it is a way of living. In this book you will find the basic recipes to start this new life full of benefits for you and yours:

1.- Simple recipes with common ingredients.

2.- Nutritional evaluation of each dish.

3.- Fun ideas for the whole family.

4.- New flavors that you must experience.

Don't wait any longer and check that it is not a fad diet, it is your new lifestyle that you have in your hands with the Plant Based Diet for Beginners.

CHAPTER 1. BREAKFAST RECIPES

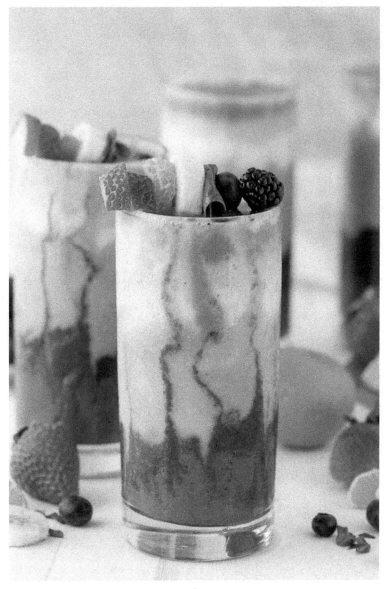

1.1 Rainbow Smoothie Pops

(Ready in about: 20-30 mins |Servings: 4 | Difficulty: Easy)

Ingredients:

Chocolate Banana Smoothie Pops:

- 1 large banana, sliced
- 3 tablespoons almond butter
- 2 tablespoons unsweetened coconut flakes
- 1 ½ cups Almond Breeze Chocolate almond milk

RED Double Berry Smoothie Pops:

- 1 ½ cups fresh or frozen sliced strawberries
- ½ cup frozen raspberries
- 1 banana, sliced
- 1 tablespoon sliced almonds
- 1 cup Almond Breeze almond milk

ORANGE Peachy Mango Smoothie Pops:

- 1 cup fresh or frozen mango cubes
- 1 cup fresh, frozen, or juice-packed peach slices

- 2 tablespoons frozen orange juice concentrate
- 1 tablespoon sliced almonds
- 1 cup Almond Breeze almond milk

YELLOW Tropical Pineapple Mango Smoothie Pops:

- 1 ½ cups fresh, frozen, or juice-packed pineapple chunks
- ⅔ cup of frozen mango cubes
- 1 tablespoon sliced almonds
- 1 tablespoon unsweetened coconut flakes

- 1 cup Almond Breeze almond milk

Super GREEN Smoothie Pops:

- 1 cup of green grapes
- 1 cup curly kale leaves
- 2 each's kiwis, peeled
- 1 tablespoon sliced almonds
- 1 cup Almond Breeze almond milk

Directions:

1. In a blender and puree, put all Ingredients until smooth. In 4-6 Popsicle moulds, pour in the puree. Add handles or mask with foil the surface of the moulds. Create carefully small

slits and place wooden sticks over each pop. Freeze for 4 hours before strong.

Nutritional Values:

NUTRITIONAL ANALYSIS PER CHOCOLATE BANANA SMOOTHIE POP:

- Calories 90

- Total Fat 3g

- Cholesterol 0mg

- Sodium 135mg

- Potassium 416mg

- Total Carbohydrate 18g

- Dietary Fibre 3g

- Sugars 8g

- Protein 2g

NUTRITIONAL ANALYSIS PER DOUBLE BERRY SMOOTHIE POP:

- Calories 140

- Total Fat 2g

- Cholesterol 0mg

- Sodium 90mg

- Potassium 306mg

- Total Carbohydrate 30g

- Dietary Fibre 7g

- Sugars 14g

- Protein 2g

NUTRITIONAL ANALYSIS PER PEACHY MANGO SMOOTHIE POP:

- Calories 100

- Total Fat 1.5

- Cholesterol 0

- Sodium 90

- Potassium 185

- Total Carbohydrate 24

- Dietary Fibre 3

- Sugars 20

- Protein 1

NUTRITIONAL ANALYSIS PER TROPICAL PINEAPPLE MANGO SMOOTHIE POP:

- Calories 130

- Total Fat 1.5g

- Cholesterol 0mg

- Sodium 90mg

- Potassium 95mg

- Total Carbohydrate 30g

- Dietary Fibre 3g

- Sugars 12g

- Protein 1g

NUTRITIONAL ANALYSIS PER SUPER GREEN SMOOTHIE POP:

- Calories 120

- Total Fat 2g

- Cholesterol 0mg

- Sodium 95mg

- Potassium 494mg

- Total Carbohydrate 25g

- Dietary Fibre 4g

- Sugars 18g

- Protein 2g

1.2 Blueberry Smoothie Bowl

(Ready in about: 10 mins |Servings: 1 | Difficulty: Easy)

Ingredients:

- 1 cup frozen blueberries
- ½ banana
- 2 tablespoons water
- 1 tablespoon cashew butter
- 1 teaspoon vanilla extract

Toppings:

- ½ banana, sliced
- 1 tablespoon sliced almonds
- 1 tablespoon unsweetened shredded coconut

Directions:

1. In the blender, mix 1/2 banana, water, cassava butter and vanilla extract into a bowl until creamy. Top banana smoothie, coconut and almonds.

Nutritional Values:

- 368.2 calories;
- protein 6.8g 14% DV;
- carbohydrates 55.4g 18% DV;
- fat 15.6g 24% DV;
- cholesterol mg;
- Sodium 8.5mg.

1.3 Citrus Healthy Smoothie

(Ready in about: 10 mins |Servings: 1 | Difficulty: Easy)

Ingredients:

- 2 each's frozen bananas, cut into small chunks
- 2 cups frozen pineapple chunks
- 1 cup fresh orange juice
- 1 cup of coconut milk
- 1 lime, juiced
- 2 teaspoons ground turmeric
- 1 (1/2 inch) piece fresh ginger, peeled and chopped
- ½ teaspoon ground nutmeg
- ice cubes as desired

Directions:

1. Blend in a blender until smooth banana, pineapple, fruit juice, cocoon milk, lime juice, turmeric and cinnamon, nutmeg and ice cubes.

Nutritional Values:

- 1234.1 calories;
- protein 11.8g 24% DV;
- carbohydrates 206g 66% DV;
- fat 51.1g 79% DV;

- cholesterol mg;

- Sodium 48.9mg 2% DV.

1.4 Energy Elixir Smoothie

(Ready in about: 10 mins |Servings: 1 | Difficulty: Easy)

Ingredients:

- 1 cup spring salad greens, or to taste

- 1 cup of frozen red grapes

- 1 chopped frozen banana

- 1 cored and chopped frozen pear

- 2 tablespoons walnuts

- water as needed

Directions:

1. In a high capacity blender, add enough water to cover. Lay greens of lettuce, red grapes, pineapple, pear and walnuts; Mix the paste to smooth and apply more water to achieve the desired consistency.

Nutritional Values:

- 420.8 calories

- protein 6.1g 12% DV;

- carbohydrates 84.7g 27% DV;

- fat 11.3g 17% DV;

- cholesterol mg;

- Sodium 27.4mg 1% DV.

1.5 Vegan Green Smoothie

(Ready in about: 5 mins | Servings: 3 | Difficulty: Easy)

Ingredients:

- 2 cups of coconut water
- 1 cup baby spinach
- 1 banana
- 6 each's sliced fresh strawberries
- 5 dates, pitted

Directions:

1. In a mixer, put together cocoon water, lettuce, bananas, strawberries and dates.

Nutritional Values:

- 118.2 calories;
- protein 2.4g 5% DV;
- carbohydrates 28.4g 9% DV;
- fat 0.7g 1% DV;
- cholesterol 0mg;
- Sodium 176.9mg 7% DV.

CHAPTER 2. QUICK ENERGY SNACKS

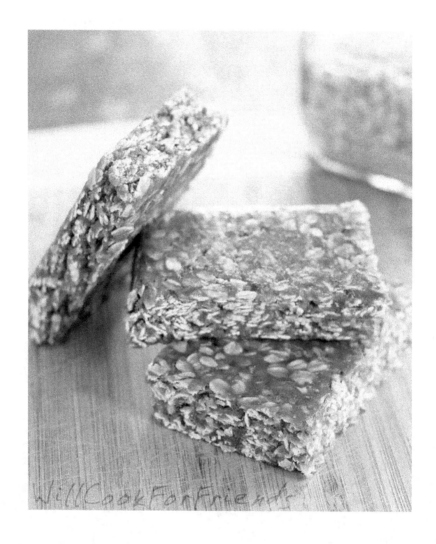

2.1 No-Bake Banana Nut Protein Bars

(Ready in about: 20 mins |Servings: 10 | Difficulty: Easy)

Ingredients:

- 9 reaches large pitted Medjool dates
- ½ cup mashed banana
- 1 teaspoon vanilla extract
- 1 cup old-fashioned rolled oats, divided
- ½ cup walnuts
- ½ cup almonds
- 2 tablespoons ground flax seed
- ¼ teaspoon ground cinnamon
- ¼ teaspoon salt
- ½ cup vanilla protein powder (such as MCT Lean®)
- ¼ cup of chocolate chips

Directions:

1. Strip an 8x8-inch pan or plastic wrap with parchment.

2. In a large food processor, mix dates, bananas and vanilla extract for around 1 minute. Stir in 3/4 flavour of walnuts, almonds, flax, cinnamon and salt; combine.

3. Crumble down the sides and add 1/4 of cup oat and protein powder left, cook for around 1 minute until the mixture is dense and well mixed. Mix the chocolate chips together.

4. Push into the jar, wet hand until even, then spoon into a prepared cup.

5. Freeze for a period of 2 to 3 hours before strong. Cut into ten squares.

Nutritional Values:

- 288.1 calories;

- protein 18.8g 38% DV;

- carbohydrates 34g 11% DV;

- fat 10.5g 16% DV;

- cholesterol 4.7mg 2% DV;

- Sodium 140.7mg 6% DV.

2.2 Protein Energy Balls

(Ready in about: 20 mins |Servings: 30 | Difficulty: Easy)

Ingredients:

- 1 cup honey

- 1 cup peanut butter

- 1 cup powdered milk

- 1 cup brown rice flour

- ½ cup coconut flour

- ½ cup rolled oats, ground
- ½ cup wheat germ
- ½ cup almonds, ground
- 1 cup hazelnuts, ground, or as needed

Directions:

1. Preheat the oven to 165 ° C (325 ° F).

2. Blend the honey, peanut butter, sugar condensed, brown grain, honey, chocolate grain, ground peas, wheat germs and ground almonds in a cup.

3. In a small dish, add ground hazelnuts. Mold the noodles into balls and roll them into ground hazelnuts. Blocks about 1 inch wide bring the balls into the baker.

4. Bake for 5 minutes in a preheated oven.

Nutritional Values:

- 172.7 calories;
- protein 5.9g 12% DV;
- carbohydrates 19.8g 6% DV;
- fat 8.9g 14% DV;
- cholesterol 0.8mg;
- Sodium 61.7mg 3% DV.

2.3 Chocolate Nutty Energy Bites

(Ready in about: 20 mins |Servings: 20 | Difficulty: Easy)

Ingredients:

- 1 cup oats
- ½ cup semi-sweet chocolate chips
- ⅓ cup chopped pecans
- ⅓ cup pumpkin seeds
- ⅓ cup chopped dried Black Mission figs
- ⅓ cup chopped dried apricots
- ¼ cup cocoa nibs
- 2 tablespoons chia seeds
- 2 tablespoons flax seeds
- ½ teaspoon pumpkin pie spice
- 1 pinch ground cardamom
- 1 cup cashew butter
- ¼ cup yacón syrup
- 2 teaspoons vanilla extract
- 1 pinch unsweetened cocoa powder, or more to taste

Directions:

1. In a big cup, add rice, chocolate nuts, nuts, pecans, pumpkin seeds, dried figs, dried apricots, cacao nibs, pumpkin pie spice and

cardamom. Apply the butter of cassava, yacón syrup and vanilla extract; mix well.

2. Place the bowl in the fridge for about 30 minutes to allow the mixture to be added. Drop the bite-sized spoonful mixture from the refrigerator onto a platter; sprinkle it with cacao powder.

Nutritional Values:

- 183 calories;

- protein 4.4g 9% DV;

- carbohydrates 16.8g 5% DV;

- fat 12g 19% DV;

- cholesterol mg;

- Sodium 6.1mg.

CHAPTER 3. RECOVERY SNACKS

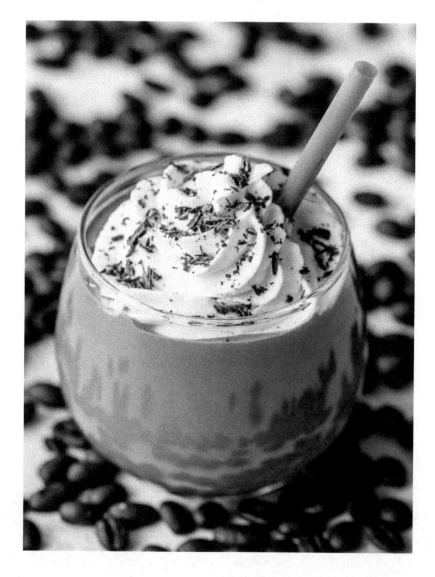

3.1 Mocha Oat Protein Shake

(Ready in about: 5 mins |Servings: 1 | Difficulty: Easy)

Ingredients:

- 1 packet carnation breakfast essentials® Rich Milk Chocolate High Protein Powder Drink Mix
- ¾ cup cold 2% milk
- ½ cup cold strong brewed coffee
- 8 each ice cubes
- ¼ cup oats

Directions:

1. In one blender, placed the mixture of cocoa, cream, coffee, ice cubes and oats. Run the mixer for 20 to 30 seconds on a smoothie loop.

Nutritional Values:

- 299.4 calories;
- protein 13.8g 28% DV;
- carbohydrates 49.3g 16% DV;
- fat 5.4g 8% DV;
- cholesterol 18.6mg 6% DV;
- Sodium 173.7mg 7% DV.

3.2 The Ultimate Toast Topping Combination

(Ready in about: 7 mins |Servings: 1 | Difficulty: Easy)

Ingredients:

- 2 slices of bread of choice
- peanut butter crunchy or creamy, whatever you like best
- 1/2 tbsp chia seeds
- 1 banana
- Honey

Directions:

1. Starting toasting two bread slices.

2. Cover a single piece of bread with the desired quantity of peanut butter after the toast.

3. Drizzle in zigzag gestures with the desired amount of sugar, relying more or less on the sweetness of the toast.

4. Sprinkle the chia seeds for both bits of toast next.

5. Then cut out a banana into 18 slices and placed it in 3 rows of 3 sections on top of your toast.

Nutritional Values:

- 572.8 calories;

- protein 23.4g 47% DV;

- carbohydrates 47.9g 16% DV;

- fat 33.4g 51% DV;

- cholesterol 283.9mg 95% DV;

- Sodium 618.7mg 25% DV.

3.3 Strawberry Banana Oatmeal Greek Yoghurt Waffles

(Ready in about: 15 mins |Servings: 2 | Difficulty: Easy)

Ingredients:

- 2 cups old-fashioned oats, gluten-free if desired

- 1 tablespoon baking powder

- 1/2 teaspoon cinnamon

- 1/4 teaspoon salt

- 1 medium ripe banana

- 1/2 cup 2% low fat plain Greek yoghurt

- 1/4 cup Almond Breeze Unsweetened Vanilla Almond milk

- 2 eggs

- 1 teaspoon vanilla extract

- 1/2 cup diced strawberries (from about 8 medium strawberries)

Directions:

1. Preheat iron and non-stick spray for the waffles.

2. Fill in all Ingredients, except strawberries, then mix properly then easily.

3. Remove the mixer and fold it softly onto strawberry with a spatula.

4. If the Belgian waffle iron is used for this, half the batter can be poured into the waffle iron and cook until the steam ends and golden-brown waffles on the outside are slightly crooked.

5. Recipe produces two waffles from Belgium. 1/2 Belgian waffle serving scale. Placed peanut butter, Greek yoghurt, berries, chia, and/or maple syrup on the top.

Nutritional Values:

- Calories: 249kcal
- Fat: 5.9g
- Saturated fat: 1.7g
- Carbohydrates: 39.4g
- Fibre: 5.5g
- Sugar: 7.1g
- Protein: 12.4g

CHAPTER 4. HIGH PROTEIN SNACKS

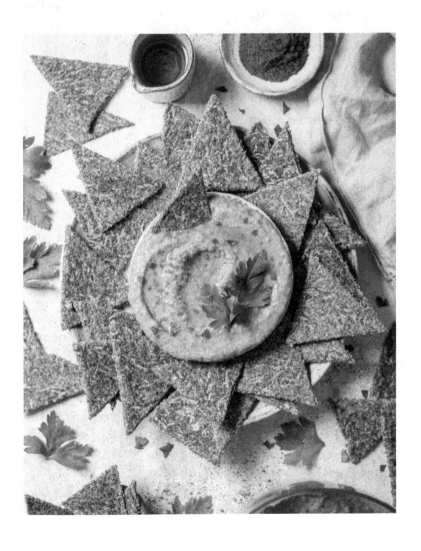

4.1 Butter Bean Dip

(Ready in about: 20 mins |Servings: 10 | Difficulty: Easy)

Ingredients:

- 1 cup butter beans (cooked)
- 1 Tbsp olive oil
- 2 Tbsp Lemon Juice
- 1/2 onion, finely chopped
- 1-2 cloves garlic, finely chopped
- Salt to taste
- 1/4 cup fresh parsley

Directions:

1. Mash the beans with butter until soft and dry.

2. Add the other elements.

3. Till well done, put together.

4. Adapt to taste (salt, fruity citrus juice, olive oil, garlic).

5. Add the olives and the cress to the decorative tub.

6. Serve with beans, maize chips or crackers of wholemeal.

Nutritional Values:

- Carbs6 g
- Dietary Fibre1 g
- Sugar0 g

- Fat4 g
- Saturated0 g
- Polyunsaturated-- g
- Monounsaturated-- g
- Trans-- g
- Protein1 g
- Sodium2 mg

- Potassium-- mg
- Cholesterol-- mg
- Vitamin A1 %
- Vitamin C19 %
- Calcium1 %
- Iron5 %

CHAPTER 5. NUTRIENT-PACKED PROTEIN SALAD RECIPES

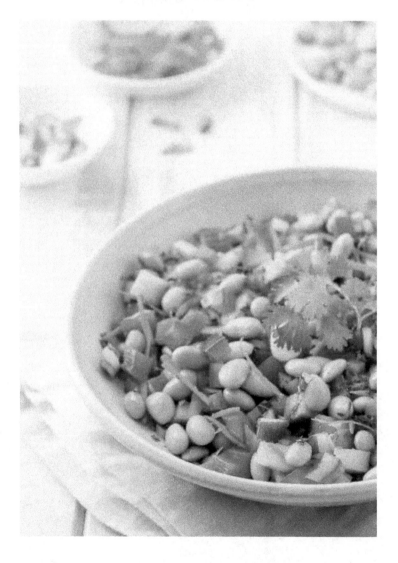

5.1 Asian Tofu & Edamame Salad

(Ready in about: 10 mins |Servings: 1 | Difficulty: Easy)

Ingredients:

- 4 cups muscling
- ½ cup shredded red cabbage
- 3 ounces baked tofu cubes
- ½ cup grated carrots
- ½ cup edamame
- ¼ cup m mandarin oranges
- One tablespoon golden raisin
- ½ cup bamboo shoots
- Two tablespoons chow Mein noodles
- Two tablespoons bottled reduced-sugar Asian sesame vinaigrette

Directions:

1. In a medium bowl, my noodles are mixed with the mezzanines muscling, cabbage, carrot, muds, grapes, raisins, and bamboo shoots. Vinaigrette drizzle.

Nutritional Values:

- 368 calories;
- total fat 11.5g 18% DV;
- saturated fat 0.5g;

- cholesterol 0mg;

- Sodium 469mg 19% DV;

- potassium -1mg;

- carbohydrates 43.5g 14% DV;

- fibre 11.5g 46% DV;

- sugar 19g;

- protein 19.5g 39% DV;

- exchange other carbs 3;

- vitamin A -1IU;

- vitamin C -1mg;

- folate -1mcg;

- calcium -1mg;

- iron -1mg;

- Magnesium -1mg.

5.2 Salmon Caesar Salad

(Ready in about: 20 mins |Servings: 4 | Difficulty: Easy)

Ingredients:

- 1 ½ tablespoon extra-virgin olive oil

- 4 (5 ounces) skinless salmon fillets (see Tip)

- One teaspoon ground pepper, divided

- ⅛ teaspoon salt plus 1/2 teaspoon, divided

- ½ cup buttermilk

- ¼ cup non-fat plain Greek yoghurt

- ¼ cup grated Parmigiano-Reggiano cheese

- Two tablespoons lemon juice

- 1 ½ teaspoon Worcestershire sauce

- One teaspoon grated garlic

- ½ teaspoon Dijon mustard

- 5 cups chopped romaine lettuce

- 3 cups chopped radicchio

- Three tablespoons thinly sliced fresh basil, plus more for garnish

- 1 ½ tablespoon chopped fresh tarragon

Directions:

1. Heat oil over a medium-high flame in a large non-stick skillet until it shines.

2. Cover 1/2 tea cubicle pepper with 1/8 tea cubicle salt. Into the pot, add the salmon and cook for three to four minutes per side until the salmon is brown and crispy. Take a plate and break into huge bits.

3. Each pepper and salt in a big bowl is well blundered with whisk buttermilk, yoghurt, from age, lemon or lime, Worcestershire, garlic, mustard & 1/2 remaining Teaspoon. Book in a little bowl 1/4 cup of sauce. Fill in

the wide bowl of cabbage, radicchio, basil and estragon and coat.

4. Place the salad on the plate and add the salmon. Serve on top with 1/4 of the cup dressing, and, if necessary, with more basil.

Nutritional Values:

- 291 calories;
- total fat 12.8g 20% DV;
- saturated fat 3.4g;
- cholesterol 73mg 24% DV;
- Sodium 575mg 23% DV;
- potassium 738mg 21% DV;
- carbohydrates 7.8g 3% DV;
- fibre 1.3g 5% DV;
- sugar 4g;
- protein 34.8g 70% DV;
- exchange other carbs 1;
- vitamin A 2281IU;
- vitamin C 26mg;
- folate 40mcg;
- calcium 242mg;
- iron 2mg;
- Magnesium 56mg.

5.3 Sweet Potato, Kale & Chicken Salad with Peanut Dressing

(Ready in about: 20-25 mins |Servings: 4 | Difficulty: Easy)

Ingredients:

- 1-pound sweet potatoes (about two medium), scrubbed and cut into 1-inch cubes
- 1 ½ teaspoon extra-virgin olive oil
- ¼ teaspoon kosher salt
- ⅛ teaspoon ground pepper
- 1/2 cup Peanut Dressing (see Associated Recipes)
- 6 cups chopped curly kale
- 2 cups shredded cooked chicken breast (see Tip)
- ¼ cup chopped unsalted peanuts

Directions:

1. Oven to 425 degrees F. Preheat. Line the rimmed sheet of the bakery with foil; lightly spray coat. Put the sweet potatoes of cabbage in a large bowl with oil, salt and pepper.

2. Place the candy on a prepared baking sheet in a single layer. Roast, turning once, about 20 minutes until tender and lightly browned and crispy outside. Before mounting bowls, put aside to cool.

3. Transfer to 4 small lidded containers two tablespoon dressing of peanut; cool for up to 4 days.

4. Divide the kale into four containers of one service (approximately 1 1/2 cups each). Top one-fourth of the sweet potatoes roasted and one-half taste of chicken. Seal up to 4 days of container and cool.

5. Throw each salad into 1 part of the dressing of peanut just before serving and cover well. Top of peanuts diced with one tablespoon.

Nutritional Values:

- 393 calories;

- total fat 15.4g 24% DV;

- saturated fat 2.7g;

- cholesterol 60mg 20% DV;

- Sodium 566mg 23% DV;

- potassium 746mg 21% DV;

- carbohydrates 31.9g 10% DV;

- fibre 5.9g 24% DV;

- sugar 8g;

- protein 30.4g 61% DV;

- exchange other carbs 2;

- vitamin A 18504IU;

- vitamin C 33mg;

- folate 59mcg;

- calcium 87mg;

- iron 2mg;

- magnesium 77mg;

- Theming; added sugar 2g.

CHAPTER 6. VEGETABLES RECIPES

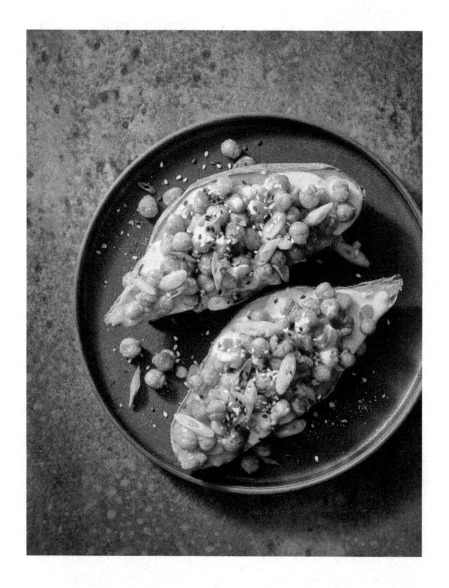

6.1 Sesame-Ginger-Chickpea-Stuffed Sweet Potatoes

(Ready in about: 20 mins |Servings: 4 | Difficulty: Easy)

Ingredients:

- Four medium sweet potatoes (about 8 oz.)

- One teaspoon canola oil

- 1 (15- oz.) can unsalted chickpeas, rinsed and drained

- Two teaspoons toasted sesame oil.

- One teaspoon garlic powder

- 1/2 teaspoon kosher salt, divided

- 1/2 teaspoon ground ginger

- Three tablespoons tahini (sesame seed paste), well stirred

- One teaspoon grated peeled fresh ginger,

- One teaspoon grated fresh garlic.

- One teaspoon rice vinegar

- Three tablespoons hot water

- Four teaspoons Sirach chilli sauce

- Two teaspoons water

- 1/4 cup thinly sliced green onions
- 1/2 teaspoon white and black sesame seeds

Directions:

1. Preheat to 400 ° F.

2. Rub canola oil in potatoes; pierce with a fork easily. For 1 hour or tender, bake at 400 ° F. Roast. Good. Break potatoes in the half longitudinal direction. Rate flesh smoothly with a button top.

3. On the bakery board, put the chickpeas, pat dry with towels of paper. Toss with sesame oil. Drain 1/4 of a teaspoon of garlic powder and ground ginger; toss. Stir after 10 minutes and bake at 400 ° F for 30 minutes.

4. Combine in cup tahini, fresh ginger and fresh garlic. Stir until looser and creamy, apply three tablespoons hot water.

5. In a bowl, mix Sirach with two tea cubes. Cover the remaining 1/4 teaspoon of salt with roughly two tahini teaspoons over every sweet potato portion. Chickpea, remaining Tahini, Sirach, green onions and sesame seeds

should be combined together.

Nutritional Values:

- Calories 413
- Fat 10.6g
- Sat fat 1.3g
- Mono fat 4.1g
- Poly fat 4.1g
- Protein 12g
- Carbohydrate 69g
- Fibre 12g
- Cholesterol 0.0mg
- Iron 3mg
- Sodium 495mg
- Calcium 136mg
- Sugars 10g
- Est. added sugars 1g

6.2 Cauliflower Gnocchi with Lemon-Caper Sauce

(Ready in about: 20 mins | Servings: 6 | Difficulty: Easy)

- 1 1/2 pounds russet potatoes (from 2 large potatoes)
- 8 cups cauliflower florets (from 1 (2 lb. 5 oz.)
- 1 cup water, divided
- 6 5/8 ounces gluten-free flour (about 1 1/4 cup), plus more for dusting
- One tablespoon olive oil

- Two tablespoons unsalted butter

- 3/4 cup unsalted vegetable stock (such as Imagine Organic)

- 1/2 teaspoon kosher salt

- 1/4 teaspoon black pepper

- Two tablespoons capers, drained and coarsely chopped.

- One teaspoon fresh lemon juice (from 1 [3 oz.] lemon)

- 1/4 cup chopped fresh parsley

- 1-ounce Parmesan cheese, grated (about 1/4 cup)

- Cooking spray

Directions:

1. Preheat to 425 ° F. Right over with a fork, poke potatoes. On a healthy microwave plate, put the potatoes; cover them with damp towels of paper. 10 to 12 minutes or tender Microwave at high. Cool down much, maybe 10 minutes. Place the cold potatoes in a large microwave-safe bowl with cauliflower and 1/2 cup of water. Place on top of high 8 to 10 min. Plastic wrap and Microwave or until soft; rinse.

2. Take cauliflower and the remaining 1/2 cup of water into a food processor. The method takes roughly 15 seconds before the mixture forms a course and broad puree.

3. Peel potatoes into a big bowl and go through the ricer. Remove the cauliflower puree until fully cooked. Add flour in batches until they are mixed to create a fluffy dough. The paste is sticky.

4. Divide dough into eight parts on a slightly blurred surface; cover it up until ready for use with a clean kitchen towel. Roll in a 3/4-inch thick rope per bit of dough. Break ropes into one-inch pieces and move them to 2 wide, spray-coated, rimmed bakeries. Clean gently with oil, the tops of gnocchi. Bake 10 to 12 minutes in a pre-heated oven, then brown on the sides. Switch to 4 bowls of service.

5. In the meantime, melt butter over medium in a medium saucepan. Oven, constantly stirring, for 2 to 3 minutes until butter becomes golden

brown. Add stock carefully and return to medium to a simmer. Simmer for about 5 minutes until the sauce is slightly reduced. Stir in the salt, pepper, capers, lemon juice and parsley and remove. In each tub, add about three tablespoons of sauce over pasta, mix it around. Parmesan dust. Serve right away.

Nutritional Values:

- Calories 290

- Fat 9g

- Sat fat 3.5g

- Unsat fat 3.6g

- Protein 10g

- Carbohydrate 49g

- Fibre 5g

- Sugars 4g

- Added sugars 0g

- Sodium 390mg

- Calcium 8% DV

- Potassium 20% DV

6.3 Stuffed Carnival Squash with Butternut Lattice

(Ready in about: 20 mins |Servings: 4 | Difficulty: Easy)

Ingredients:

- 6 ounces sourdough bread, cut into 1/2-inch pieces

- Two tablespoons unsalted butter

- One tablespoon olive oil, divided

- 1 1/2 cups pre-chopped fresh onion, carrot and celery mix

- Two teaspoons chopped fresh sage.

- 1 cup unsalted vegetable stock

- 2 large eggs

- Three tablespoons chopped flat-leaf parsley.

- 3/4 teaspoon kosher salt, divided

- 1/2 teaspoon ground black pepper

- 4 (16- oz.) small carnival squash or acorn squash

- One medium, long butternut squash

- One teaspoon honey

Directions:

1. Oven to 400 ° C.

2. Onto the rimmed bakery put the bread cubes on. Bake 15-20 minutes at 400 ° or stirring once until golden brown. Remove from the oven and cool for 5 minutes.

3. Place butter and 1 1/2 teaspoon oil on a medium-hot skillet. Apply the onion and the wise to pan; stir regularly simmers for 4-5 minutes or

tenderly. Let it down. Stir in a medium bowl with a whisk and blend with the stock and the eggs. Add the flour, ointment blend, dogs, 1/2 teaspoon salt and pepper; powder and let set and for 10 minutes, or for 5 minutes, until the liquid has been absorbed.

4. Split the top 1/4 from squash carnival. Scrap seeds and pith with a spoon, leave a 3/4 "bottom of the squash. Remove the thin slice from the squash bottom such that they lie smooth and dry. Break the bread mix for

squash equally. Placed on a bakery sheet lined with the paper of parchment. When pierced with a sharp knife, cook at 400 ° for 35 minutes or tenderly.

5. Cut whole neck squash from the bulb as squash bakes, reserving bulbs for further use. Break your neck half longitudinally; save half for another day. Place the remainder of the neck on the cutting board part, cut side down. Split into 1/8 "slabs. Longitudinally. Remove the ribbons from either side of the

platter using a vegetable peeler.

6. In a shallow cup, mix the remaining 11/2 teaspoons of oil with butter. Placed on a cutting board or work surface 12 squash b and (6 horizontal lines and six vertical strips). Mind creating four lattice tops three more times. Using a fish spatula or a thin metal spatula to remove the grating after you have cooked until the squash is tender. The overhang weighs about 1 inch with the scissors. Clean the grille with the combination of honey. Load the remaining 1/2 teaspoon of salt onto the grill generously. Bake 10 minutes at 400 ° C.

Nutritional Values:

- Calories 450

- Fat 13g

- Sat fat 5g

- Mono fat 5g

- Protein 13g

- Carbohydrates 78g

- Fibre 10g

- Sugars 15g

- Sodium 749mg

CHAPTER 7. STAPLE LUNCH RECIPES

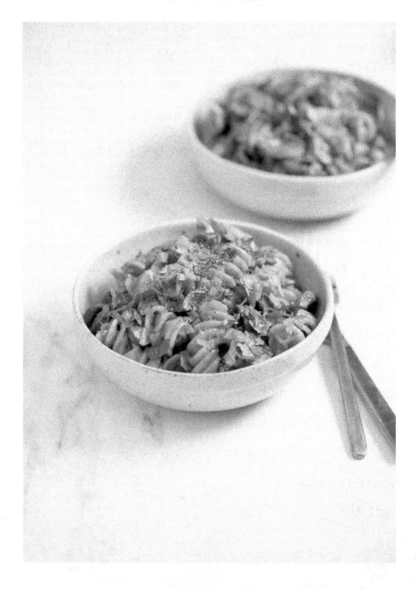

7.1 One-Pot Vegan Mushroom Stroganoff

(Ready in about: 15 mins |Servings: 4 | Difficulty: Easy)

Ingredients:

- 1 small yellow onion, sliced and quartered

- 10 ounces (280 g) criminal mushrooms, cut in half or fourths

- 8 ounces (225 g) dry rotini pasta*; about 4 cups

- 4 cups *imitation* "beef-flavoured" broth (or sub vegetable broth)

- 2 tablespoons nutritional yeast

- 1/4 teaspoon freshly ground black pepper, plus more to taste

- 1/3 cup (85 g) cashew butter*

- 1 tablespoon lemon juice

- 1/4 - 1/2 teaspoon kosher salt (*optional*)

- 2 tablespoons parsley, chopped

Directions:

1. Sauté the Onion: to a big pot over medium heat, add 1/4 of a cup (60 ml) of water. Slice the oreganos and fry, roughly 3 to 5 minutes, until translucent. Even

51

if you like, the onions can be sautéed in 1 tablespoon instead of water.

2. Cook the pasta: add spaghetti, champagne, beef-flavoured soup, food yeast and black pepper to prepare. Bring to a boil over high temperature, then reduce heat to medium-low and cook for 10-15 minutes, mixing from time to time to make sure the pan is not oily.

3. Get this moist. Turn off the heat and then apply the cake butter and lemon juice to the mix. Check the pasta, and, if necessary, add additional salt.

4. Serve: top with chopped fresh pepper and parsley and eat soft. Eat. Place remainders for up to one week in the refrigerator in an airtight jar.

Nutritional Values:

- Calories313%

- Daily Value*

- Total Fat 1.5g2%

- Cholesterol 0mg0%

- Sodium 1286.8mg56%

- Total Carbohydrate 55g20%

- Sugars 4.2g

- Protein 14.9g30%

- Vitamin A7%

- Vitamin C27%

7.2 Roasted Red Pepper Pasta

(Ready in about: 15 mins |Servings: 2-4 | Difficulty: Easy)

Ingredients:

- 8 ounces (230 g) pasta of choice

- 8.5 ounces (240 g) roasted red peppers*, drained and rinsed if using canned

- 2 cloves garlic

- 1 cup (235 ml) full-fat coconut milk

- ½ cup (115 ml) vegetable broth

(homemade or store-bought)

- 1/4 tsp red chilli flakes (optional)

Directions:

1. Carry a big pot of salted brings to the boil, then cook the pasta as instructed in the packet.

2. Meanwhile, add the tomatoes, ginger, chocolate powder, brown vegetables and optional red pickles to the mixer. Mix high up until sauce is thick and smooth for 40 - 60 seconds. When required, season with

pepper and salt to taste.

3. When baked, drain the sauce, but not rinse. Top up the stove and put the red pepper sauce back into the empty tank. Cook the sauce for 2 to 3 minutes, until bubbly and thickened and serve it over medium to high heat.

4. Apply the paste to the pot and then smash it with a spoon or tongs. When it seems like the sauce is runny, let the pasta stay for 3 to 5 minutes more to soak.

5. Move the pasta to the cups, then top as you wish.

Nutritional Values:

- Calories170.2

- Total Fat4.4 g

- Saturated Fat1.4 g

- Polyunsaturated Fat0.6 g

- Monounsaturated Fat2.2 g

- Cholesterol3.9 mg

- Sodium336.9 mg

- Potassium117.8 mg

- Total Carbohydrate27.4 g

- Dietary Fibre4.4 g

- Sugars2.8 g

- Protein6.7 g

7.3 South-Western Black Bean Casserole

(Ready in about: 20 mins |Servings: 4-6 | Difficulty: Easy)

Ingredients:

- 1 3/4 cups (415 ml) low-Sodium vegetable broth **(homemade or store-bought)**
- 1 cup (~ 250 g) chunky salsa
- 2 tablespoons nutritional yeast
- 1 red bell pepper, diced
- 1 green bell pepper, diced
- 1/2 yellow onion, diced
- 2 cans (510 g) canned black beans, drained and rinsed; about 2 3/4 cups
- 1 cup (182 g) uncooked brown rice
- 1/2 bunch cilantro leaves, chopped
- **Optional toppings: Chipotle Mayo**, avocado, fresh tomatoes.

Directions:

1. Preheat to 400F. In a medium kettle, blend the vegetables broth, salsa and nuts' yeast to cook.

2. When the liquid heats up, peppers and oreganos scatter uniformly into a kettle or saucepan. Spread over the vegetables with the black beans and put rice over.

3. Take the vegetable broth off the heat until its boiling and spread it generously over the saucepan. Cover the saucepan with aluminium film (or parchment paper, aluminium foil followed) and steam for 60 minutes in the centre rack of the oven.

4. Take fresh coriander, avocado, or chipotle mayo from of the oven and top (or serve as requested). Cool the residual leftovers up to a week in a filtered fridge, or up to a month in a freezer.

Nutritional Values:

- Calories Per Serving: 303

- 12%Total Fat 9.4g

- 14%Cholesterol 43.2mg

- 20%Sodium 465.3mg

- 12%Total Carbohydrate 32.6g

- 37%Dietary Fibre 10.3g

- Sugars 5.3g

- 47%Protein 23.5g

- 9%Vitamin A 79.9µg

- 42%Vitamin C 37.6mg

CHAPTER 8. SAUCES
RECIPES

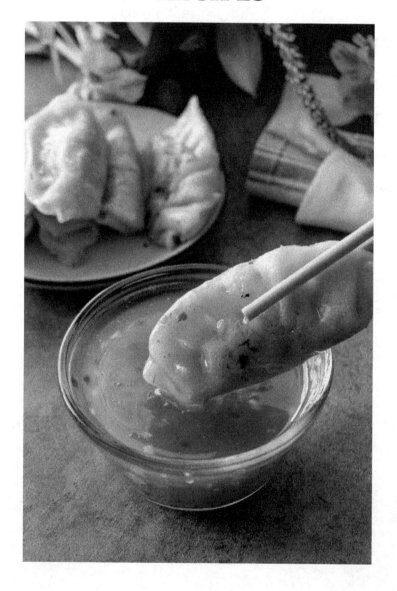

8.1 Easy Asian Dipping Sauce

(Ready in about: 15 mins |Servings: 2 | Difficulty: Easy)

Ingredients:

- 1 tablespoon and 1 teaspoon soy sauce

- 1 tablespoon and 1 teaspoon rice wine vinegar

- 1 teaspoon honey

- 1/2 clove minced garlic

- 1 teaspoon minced fresh ginger root

- 1/4 teaspoon sesame seeds

- 1/4 teaspoon sesame oil

Directions:

1. In a cup, mix the soy sauce together, sugar, butter, garlic, ginger, sesame seeds, and sesame oil.

Nutritional Values:

- 28.1 calories;

- protein 0.8g 2% DV;

- carbohydrates 4.2g 1% DV;

- fat 1.1g 2% DV;

- cholesterol 0mg;

- Sodium 601.7mg 24% DV.

8.2 Béarnaise Sauce

(Ready in about: 5 mins |Servings: 2 | Difficulty: Easy)

Ingredients:

- 2 teaspoons dried tarragon
- 1/4 cup red wine vinegar
- 2 teaspoons minced shallots
- 1 egg yolks
- 1 tablespoon and 1 teaspoon hot water
- 1/8 lemon, juiced
- 3/8 pinch salt
- 3/8 pinch cayenne pepper
- 1/3 cup butter, melted

Directions:

1. In a big bowl, hop tarragon, wine vinegar and shallot diced for 10 to 15 minutes over medium heat or until the mixture is paste-like. Take it out of the sun.

2. In the double boiler, set over a simmering water mix egg yolk, 1/8 cup warm water, lemon juice, salt and pepper. Cook and extract before the mixture reach mayonnaise consistency. Take out the hot combination. Stirring constantly,

slowly add the molten butter. If the mixture is so thick, the remainder is 1/8 cup hot water fine. Apply the mixture of tarragon, sugar, vinegar, and shallot and blend properly.

Nutritional Values:

- 308.7 calories;
- protein 2.3g 5% DV;
- carbohydrates 2.9g 1% DV;
- fat 33g 51% DV;
- cholesterol 183.8mg 61% DV;
- Sodium 226.9mg 9% DV.

8.3 Sambal Sauce

(Ready in about: 20 mins |Servings: 2 | Difficulty: Easy)

Ingredients:

- 2 tablespoons chopped serrano chills, with seeds
- 3/4 teaspoon white sugar
- 3/4 teaspoon salt
- 1/2 teaspoon beacon shrimp paste
- 1/8 tomato, chopped
- 1/8 onion, chopped
- 1/8 bulb garlic, peeled and crushed
- 3/4 teaspoon fresh lime juice

- 3/4 teaspoon vegetable oil

- 1/4 lemongrass, bruised

- 1/4 fresh curry leaves

- 1/8 (1/2 inch) piece galangal, thinly sliced

- 3/4 teaspoon tamarind juice

Directions:

1. Put serrano's potatoes in a blender and mix until smooth, adding sugar, salt, pulp, tomato, onion, and garlic and lime juice. Heat a medium-high heat vegetable oil in a sprinkler. Add the lemongrass, curry leaves and galangal in chilli puree. Cook and combine before colour improves, around 15 minutes and become very odorous. Connect the tamarind juice and simmer for another 1 minute. Strain before serving.

Nutritional Values:

- 38.1 calories;

- protein 0.7g 1% DV;

- carbohydrates 5.4g 2% DV;

- fat 1.8g 3% DV;

- cholesterol 0.6mg;

- Sodium 875mg 35% DV.

8.4 Chef John's Tzatziki Sauce

(Ready in about: 20 mins |Servings: 2 | Difficulty: Easy)

Ingredients:

- 1/8 large English cucumber, peeled and grated
- 1/8 teaspoon salt
- 1/3 cup Greek yoghurt
- 5/8 clove garlic, minced
- 1/8 pinch cayenne pepper for garnish
- 1/8 lemon, juiced
- 1/8 sprig fresh dill for garnish
- 1/8 teaspoon chopped fresh mint
- 1/8 teaspoon salt
- 1/8 sprig fresh dill for garnish
- 1/8 pinch cayenne pepper for garnish

Directions:

1. Sprinkle the rusty cucumber in a bowl with two teaspoons salt and give 10 to 15 minutes for juice to be produced.

2. In a separate tub, put yoghurt. Dump cucumber and its juice on a thick, dry towel of paper or cloth and extract from the cucumber the full

amount of moisture. In milk, blend cucumber. Stir in a complete blend of garlic, cayenne pepper and citrus fruit juice.

3. Add salt and black pepper in the mixture of yoghurt/cucumber. Adapt to taste single seasoning.

4. Plastic bowl cover and freeze for three or four hours (or overnight). Refrigerate. Switch to a serving bowl and fill with dill and cayenne pepper sprinkle for flavor.

Nutritional Values:

- 48.5 calories;

- protein 2.2g 5% DV;

- carbohydrates 2.5g 1% DV;

- fat 3.4g 5% DV;

- cholesterol 7.5mg 3% DV;

- Sodium 119.6mg 5% DV.

8.5 Alfredo Sauce

(Ready in about: 20 mins |Servings: 2 | Difficulty: Easy)

Ingredients:

- 2 tablespoons butter

- 1/2 cup heavy cream

- 1/2 clove garlic, crushed

- 1/2 cup and 1 tablespoon and 2 teaspoons freshly grated Parmesan cheese
- 2 tablespoons chopped fresh parsley

Directions:

In a medium saucepan, melt the butter over low temperature. Stir in the milk and boil for five minutes and then add garlic and cheese. Mix in the hot pepper and eat.

Nutritional Values:

- 438.8 calories;
- protein 13g 26% DV;
- carbohydrates 3.4g 1% DV;
- fat 42.1g 65% DV;
- cholesterol 138.4mg 46% DV;
- Sodium 565.3mg 23% DV.

CHAPTER 9. GRAINS AND BEANS RECIPES

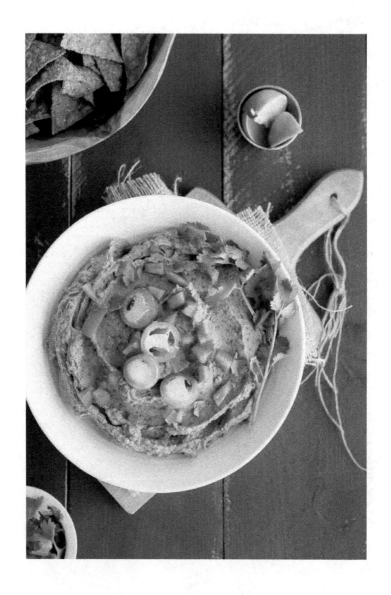

9.1 Creamy Black Bean Avocado Dip

(Ready in about: 5 mins |Servings: 4 | Difficulty: Easy)

Ingredients

- 15 oz. can black beans
- One avocado
- 1/2 cup salsa
- 3 Tbsp. water
- One clove garlic (minced)
- 3/4 tsp. cumin
- 1/8 tsp. salt (more to taste)

Other additions (optional):

- Nutritional yeast, chipotle, cilantro, lime, jalapeno, cayenne, etc.

Directions:

1. Rinse the black beans and rinse them. Reserve nearly 1/2 cup of the beans.

2. in a blender or food processor, but the rest of the beans and all other ingredients.

3. Mix before the perfect texture * is achieved. Excellent

seasonings and change as desired.

4. Throw the remainder of the black beans into a bowl and combine.

5. If you prefer, garnish with cilantro, food yeast, etc.

6. Tell me, hot, cold, or temperate space!

Nutritional Values:

- Calories: 153kcal

- carbohydrates: 20g

- protein: 7g

- fat: 6g

- saturated fat: 1g

- potassium: 544mg

- fibre: 9g

- sugar: 1g

- vitamin A: 183 IU

- vitamin C: 7mg

- calcium: 49mg

- iron: 2mg

9.2 Black Bean Brownies

(Ready in about: 20 mins | Servings: 4 | Difficulty: Easy)

Ingredients:

- 15 ounces <u>black beans, drained and rinsed</u>

- Two whole bananas

- ⅓ cup <u>agave nectar</u>

- ¼ cup <u>unsweetene d cocoa</u>

- 1 tbsp <u>cinnamon</u>

- 1 tsp <u>vanilla extract</u>

- ¼ cup <u>raw sugar</u> (optional)

- ¼ cup <u>instant oats</u>

Directions:

1. Preheat oven to 350 F. Grease an 8x8" pan and set aside. Combine all ingredients, except oats, in a food processor or blender and blend until smooth, scraping sides as needed. Stir in the oats and pour batter into the pan. Bake approximately 30 minutes or until a toothpick inserted in the centre comes out clean. Allow cooling before slicing. Chef's Note: if you find these brownies are too soft or too fudge-y, add another 1/4 cup oats or flour.

Nutritional Values:

- Calories: 112

- Fat: 0.90g

- Carbohydrate: 24.70g

- Dietary Fibre: 4.80g

- Sugars: 12.20g

- Protein: 3.50g

9.3 Uptown Cowboy Caviar

(Ready in about: 20 mins |Servings: 10 | Difficult: Easy)

Ingredients:

- (15 ounces) can black beans, rinsed and drained
- 1 (15 ounces) can black-eyed peas, rinsed and drained
- 1 (15 ounces) can pinto beans, rinsed and drained
- 1 (11 ounces) can yellow shoe peg corn, drained
- 1 cup diced celery
- 1 small bunch cilantro leaves, chopped
- ½ red bell pepper, diced
- ½ yellow bell pepper, diced
- ½ cup chopped green onion
- 1 (2 ounces) jar chopped pimento peppers
- 2 tablespoons minced jalapeno pepper
- 1 tablespoon minced garlic
- ½ cup of rice vinegar
- ½ cup extra virgin olive oil
- ⅓ cup white sugar
- 1 teaspoon salt

70

- ½ teaspoon ground black pepper

Directions:

1. In a large pot, mix dark beans, pinto peppers, shoe peg maize, celery, bell pepper, red and purple, green onion, pimento peppers, jalapeno pepper and garlic. Set aside.

2. Cook in a saucepan, over medium to high heat, rice vinegar, olive oil, sugar, salt and black pepper until the sugar is absorbed, around five minutes. Cool all at room temperature and spill over the mixture of the beans. Cover and cool for two or overnight hours. Drain before eating.

Nutritional Values:

- 265.8 calories;

- protein 7.2g 15% DV;

- carbohydrates 32.6g 11% DV;

- fat 12.1g 19% DV;

- cholesterol 0mg;

- Sodium 709.9mg 28% DV.

9.4 Mississippi Caviar

(Ready in about: 15 mins |Servings: 6 | Difficulty: Easy)

Ingredients:

- 1 (15.25 ounce) can whole kernel corn, drained

- 1 (15 ounces) can black beans, rinsed and drained

- 1 (10 ounces) can diced tomatoes and green chillies, drained

- One avocado, cut into 1/2-inch chunks

- 1 Roma (plum) tomato, chopped - or more to taste

- 1 small red onion, chopped

- 3 tablespoons pickled jalapeno pepper rings, finely minced

- ½ cup Italian-style salad dressing, or more to taste

- salt and black pepper to taste

- hot pepper sauce to taste

Directions:

1. Mix peas, black beans, canned tomatoes and chillies together in a big bowl, avocados, Roma tomato, onion, carrots, jalapenos and salads together. Add salt, pepper and hot pepper sauce to taste. Cool before serving.

Nutritional Values:

- 183.6 calories;

- protein 3.2g 7% DV;

- carbohydrates 21.9g 7% DV;

- fat 11.2g 17% DV;

- cholesterol 0 mg;

- Sodium 762.6mg 31% DV

CHAPTER 10. PLANT-BASED DIET FOR SOME MINOR HEALTH ISSUES

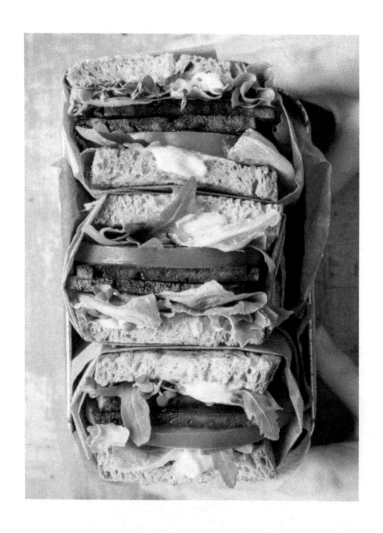

10.1 Vegan BLT Sandwich

(Ready in about: 15 mins |Servings: 1 | Difficulty: Easy)

Ingredients:

PER SANDWICH

- Two slices eureka! whole-grain bread
- One medium ripe avocado
- Salt, to taste
- ¼ cup coconut bacon
- One medium ripe red tomato
- Freshly ground black pepper
- Several small leaves of romaine or butter lettuce
- Two slices eureka! whole-grain bread
- One medium ripe avocado
- Salt, to taste
- ¼ cup coconut bacon
- One medium ripe red tomato
- Freshly ground black pepper
- Several small leaves of romaine or butter lettuce

Directions:

1. Before you go to the sandwich, make sure

you make the coconut bacon (it is easy to make, and you will have plenty of remains that will be frozen well). When you are ready to make sandwiches, toast your desired doneness first with bread.

2. Cut the avocado halfway and push the flesh of the avocado into a bowl. Add a little salt and smoothly and quickly stretch the avocado with a fork. Taste, if necessary, and add additional salt.

3. Spread the avocado over each bread slice. Put the coconut bacon heavily on a toast and press into the avocado lightly to help stick.

4. Slice the tomato into one and a half slices. Sprinkle with black pepper and top with bacon toast 2 to 3 pieces of tomato. Put the rest of the tomatoes on top, side down and add lettuce to it. Cut the sandwich half with a tightened knife if you prefer.

Nutritional values:

- Calories 637

- Total Fat 69.8g 90%

- Saturated Fat 6g

- Trans Fat 0g

- Polyunsaturated Fat 7.2g

- Monounsaturated Fat 16.8g 0%

- Cholesterol 0mg 0%

- Sodium 993.9mg 43%

- Total Carbohydrate 58.5g 21%

- Dietary Fibre 26.5g 95%

- Sugars 19.1g

- Protein 17.4g 35%

10.2 Tomato, Peach & Avocado Bruschetta

(Ready in about: 5 mins | Servings: 4-6 | Difficulty: Easy)

Ingredients:

- 1 cup sliced cherry tomatoes

- a drizzle of olive oil

- 1 garlic clove, minced

- a drizzle of white balsamic vinegar

- 2-4 peaches, cut into small pieces

- 1 avocado, diced
- chopped basil and/or mint
- generous amounts of salt & pepper
- about 4 - 6 slices of bread

Directions:

1. In a small cup, place tomatoes with olive oil, white balsamic, hairy garlic, salt, and pepper.

2. In addition, add pike, avocado, basil, and mint. Add salt and pepper to taste and change seasoning.

3. Toast bread slices and layer them all together. Drizzle and serve directly with more olive oil.

Nutritional Values:

- Calories: 400
- Saturated fat: 0g
- Cholesterol: 0mg
- Sodium: 0mg
- Carbohydrates: 0g
- Fibre: 0g
- Sugar: 0g
- Protein: 0g

10.3 Kiwi Avocado Salsa Verde

(Ready in about: 10 mins |Servings: 2 | Difficulty: Easy)

Ingredients:

- kiwi, peeled and diced

- scallions, chopped

- 1 avocado, diced

- ½ cup chopped cilantro

- ¼ cup chopped red onion* (see note)

- juice and zest of 1 to 2 limes (about 2 tablespoons of juice)

- 1 garlic clove, minced

- 1 jalapeño pepper, thinly sliced (optional)

- sea salt

- Garden of Eating' White Corn Bowls

Directions:

1. Mix kiwi and jalapeño in a little cup, if you are using, with a generous pinch of salt from the sea and cilantro, onion, lime, and zest juice. Additional salt and/or lime juice are tasted in season. Serve with White Corn Bowls Garden of Feeding.

Nutritional values:

- Calories 81 kcal 4%

- Fat 5.6g 9%

- Saturated fat 0.8g 4%

- Carbs 8.8g 3%

- Sodium 6mg<1%

- 2.9g sugar

- 3.8g fibre

- 1.2g protein

- 0mg cholesterol

10.4 Avocado Basil Cucumber Bites

(Ready in about: 10 mins |Servings: 4 | Difficulty: Easy)

Ingredients:

- 1 ripe avocado, peeled and pitted

- ½ cup fresh basil leaves

- 1 tablespoon lime juice

- 1 clove garlic

- ¼ teaspoon salt

- ¼ teaspoon ground black pepper

- 1 cucumber, cut into 1/4-inch slices

- 1 plum tomato, cut into 1/4-inch slices

- 1 tablespoon plain yoghurt, or to taste

Directions:

1. In a food processor or mix until smooth, add avocado, basil, lime, garlic, salt, and pepper.

2. Break the mixture of tomato and yoghurt on each piece of peanut and cover of tomato.

Nutritional values:

- 96.7 Calories;
- Protein 1.9g 4% Dv;
- Carbohydrates 7.8g 3% Dv;
- Fat 7.6g 12% Dv;
- Cholesterol 0.2mg;
- Sodium 153.8mg 6% Dv.

CHAPTER 11. PLANT-BASED

FOR HEALTHY EYES

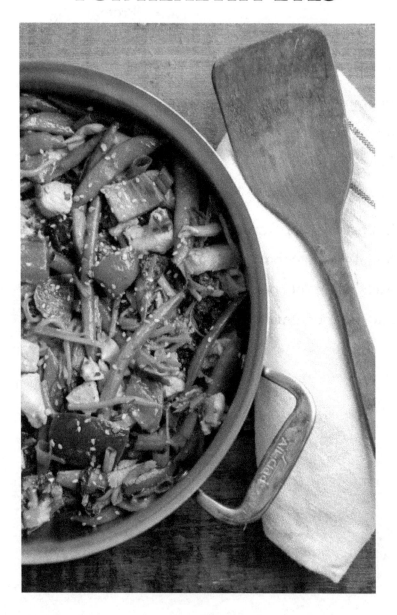

11.1 Vegetable Stir Fry with Orange Sauce

(Ready in about: 25-30 mins |Servings: 4 | Difficulty: Easy)

Ingredients:

FOR THE BROWN RICE

- cups uncooked brown rice (336g)
- cups water (945 ml)
- One tablespoon butter (14g)

FOR THE ORANGE SAUCE

- 3/4 cup reduced-sodium soy sauce (177 ml)
- 1/2 cup orange juice (120 ml)
- Two tablespoons corn-starch (20g)
- Two tablespoons orange zest
- Four teaspoons sugar (17g)

FOR THE STIR FRY

- 1/4 cup light olive oil (60 ml)
- cups red bell pepper, cut in 1-inch slices (295g)
- 2 cups carrots, peeled and cut in thin diagonal slices (270g)
- 3 cups broccoli florets (190g)

- One green onion, cut in 1-inch diagonal slices (45g)

- Two zucchinis, sliced in 1/4-inch coins (500g)

- 1/4 teaspoon sesame seeds, for garnish

Directions:

COOKING THE RICE

1. In a 2-quarter kettle, place the bath, cover and simmer. Add salt until dissolved, blend in rice and reduce to medium-low heat. Cook the lid askew for 35 minutes, or to collect all the water.

2. Take the pot from the heat for 5 minutes, let it rest. Stir in 2 teaspoons of sugar, fluffing the rice with a fork.

MAKING THE ORANGE SAUCE

1. In a small cup, mix soy sauce, orange juice, maize starch and sugar together.

COOKING THE STIR FRY

1. Heat oil over high heat in two large bowls or a wok. Stirring vigorously, add carrots and simmer for about 2 minutes. Cook for 6 minutes the remainder of the vegetables. Stir always, so they don't

burn when you like vegetables to pass.

2. Sprinkle the orange sauce with the maize settling down in the dish. Create a vacuum and put the sauce into space in the centre of the vegetables. Enable it to bubble for a few seconds and thicken.

3. Mix the orange sauce in and cook for 1 minute while mixing continuously.

4. Using the warm brown rice to stir fry sweet. Sprinkle with sesame seeds. Garnish.

Nutritional Values:

- Calories 618

- Total Fat 20.7g 27%

- Cholesterol 7.5mg 3%

- Sodium 1817.4mg 79%

- Total Carbohydrate 98.5g 36%

- Dietary Fibre 9.7g 34%

- Sugars 15.1g

- Protein 15.8g 32%

11.2 Orange Cauliflower–A Vegetarian's Orange Chicken

(Ready in about: 20 mins |Servings: 2 | Difficulty: Easy)

Ingredients

- One medium-sized cauliflower is broken

into florets (made approx. 3 cups)

- 1/2 cup diced bell peppers (Mixed colours)

- 1/3 cup + 2 tbsp corn starch

- 1/2 cup all-purpose flour (Maida)

- 1/4 to 1/2 cup water (to make a batter)

- Oil for frying + 1 tbsp

- Two cloves garlic, minced

- 1/4 teaspoon ground ginger

- One tablespoon orange zest

- 3/4 cup vegetable broth

- 1/2 cup freshly squeezed orange juice

- tsp soy sauce

- tbsp sugar

- 1 tsp Sirach (Or any other red chilli paste/sauce)

- 1/4 teaspoon crushed black pepper

- Salt to taste

- 1/2 teaspoon sesame seeds

- 2 tbsp green onion, thinly sliced

Directions:

1. Heat oil in a frying pan.

2. Heat half a tbsp in another cup. Add oil and peppers. Oil and

extract. Salt them for a minute or two before they become white. Be sure the peppers don't overcook. Only quit it as soon as it's over.

3. Mix the maize starch with the whole-use flour to produce a smooth batter with a salt and water pinch.

4. The batter should be as dense as possible to cover the cauliflower seeds uniformly.

5. Top into the batter and place in hot oil for frying each floret of cauliflower. Fry it in batches so that the pan doesn't get overfilled.

6. When the batter is fluffy, wash it out of the oil and put it on paper towels.

7. When all the Flores have been cooked, you have to keep them crisp before you are prepared to sprinkle them in the sauce. You can either keep them warm in a pre-heated oven or fried them again in hot oil for a minute before you apply the sauce.

8. In the pan, the peppers were roasted in heat 1/2 tbsp oil for the sauce. Connect the ginger and garlic minced.

9. Sauté them before they become golden for a minute. Fill in the orange peel.

10. Add the broth, raspberry, Sirach, soy, sugar and combine well.

11. In the meanwhile, blend with water 2 tbsp of maize starch to produce a thin paste.

12. After the mixture of broth and orange starts to simmer, reduce the heat. Incorporate salt and crushed black pepper (if necessary)

13. In a slow, steady stream, apply the maize starch paste to the boiling mix. Make sure you still stir with your other hand before applying maize flour paste to the simmering mixture.

14. Thickening the mixture, put the cauliflower and bell pepper in the fried cauliflower.

15. Mix well and add a little fire for a minute or two, sun.

16. Switch to a serving platter and decorate with sesame seeds and olive oreganos.

Nutritional Values:

- Calories 469

- Fat 6g

- Carbs 90g

- Fibre 6g

- Sugar 23g

11.3 Avocado and Orange Sandwich

(Ready in about: 10 mins |Servings: 4 | Difficulty: Easy)

Ingredients:

- 8 (1 ounce) slices whole-wheat bread

- 1 large navel orange, peeled and cut into 1/4-inch thick slices

- 2 large avocados - peeled, pitted and sliced

- 1 (5 ounces) package alfalfa sprouts

- 2 teaspoons balsamic vinaigrette

Directions:

1. Place four slices of bread on a flat surface; put two slices of lime, even quantities of avocados slices and even various sprouts on top of each slice. Put 1 tablespoon of balsamic vinaigrette through each sandwich. Fix bread slices on top of each and enjoy.

Nutritional Values:

- 407.1 calories;

- protein 12g 24% DV;

- carbohydrates 42.6g 14% DV;
- fat 23.7g 37% DV;
- cholesterol mg;
- Sodium 309mg 12% DV.

CHAPTER 12. PLANT-BASED DIET FOR HEALTHY IMMUNE SYSTEM

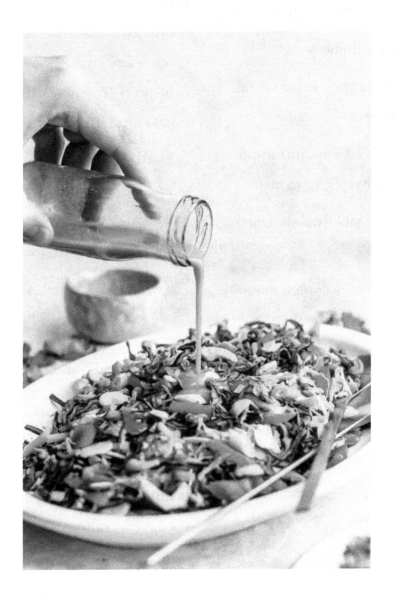

12.1 Ginger Salad Dressing

(Ready in about: 5 mins |Servings: 3 | Difficulty: Easy)

Ingredients:

- ½ cup extra-virgin olive oil

- Two tablespoons apple cider vinegar, to taste

- Two tablespoons Dijon mustard

- One tablespoon maple syrup or honey, to taste

- Two teaspoons finely grated fresh ginger

- ½ teaspoon fine sea salt

- About 20 twists of freshly ground black pepper

Directions:

1. Place all the ingredients in a container or small bowl until thoroughly combined. Often it takes a few minutes to heat up if the mustard is cold until it absorbs.

2. Shake and if desired, adjust — add another teaspoon of apple cider vinegar or add a teaspoon of maple syrup (I normally add one). For more sweetness, add another teaspoon or two.

3. The dressing in the salad would remain healthy for ten days in the refrigerator. True

olive oil will solidify slightly if cold; if so, just let it warm in a microwave-secure jar and microwave it for just 15 to 30 seconds, to room temperature for a couple of minutes.

Nutritional Values:

- Calories 88
- Total Fat 9.3g 12%
- Saturated Fat 1.3g
- Trans Fat 0g
- Polyunsaturated Fat 1g
- Monounsaturated Fat 6.7g 0%
- Cholesterol 0mg 0%
- Sodium 153.7mg 7%
- Total Carbohydrate 1.3g 0%
- Dietary Fibre 0g 0%
- Sugars 1g
- Protein 0g 0%

12.2 Pomegranate & Pear Green Salad with Ginger Dressing

(Ready in about: 20-30 mins |Servings: 6 | Difficulty: Easy)

Ingredients:

Salad

- ½ cup raw pecans (halves or pieces)
- 5 ounces baby arugula

- 2 ounces (about ½ cup) goat cheese or feta, crumbled
- One large ripe Bartlett pear, thinly sliced
- 1 Honey crisp or Gala apple, thinly sliced
- Arils from 1 pomegranate

Ginger dressing

- ¼ cup extra-virgin olive oil
- One tablespoon apple cider vinegar, to taste
- One tablespoon Dijon mustard
- One tablespoon maple syrup or honey
- One teaspoon finely grated fresh ginger
- ¼ teaspoon fine sea salt
- About ten twists of freshly ground black pepper

Directions:

1. Put them in a pot for medium heat, toast the pecans. Taste, mix, regularly mix, about 4 to 5 minutes, until they are fragrant and golden on the outside. Remove the pecan from heat and cut it roughly (if you started with pecan bits, you should not cut them off). Place aside. Set aside.

2. Place the arugula over a large serving dish (or tub, but the

salad looks more stunning on a plate). Sprinkle over the arugula with sliced pecans and split chives. Remove the pear and apple slices and put them in sections around the salad. New grenade arils scatter in.

3. Combine all the ingredients and whisk until mixed for preparation of the sauce. Smell and apply another tea cubicle of vinegar if it isn't yet zippy enough.

4. Wait until the dressing is done (the dressing is full time turning greens) when you are able to wear the ginger loosely in the salad (maybe you don't need it all). Serve easily. Serve promptly.

Nutritional Values:

- Calories 253

- Total Fat 18.1g 23%

- Saturated Fat 3.3g

- Trans Fat 0g

- Polyunsaturated Fat 3g

- Monounsaturated Fat 10.5g 0%

- Cholesterol 4.4mg 1%

- Sodium 200.8mg 9%

- Total Carbohydrate 21.8g 8%

- Dietary Fibre 4.7g 17%

- Sugars 15.3g

- Protein 4.1g 8%

CHAPTER 13. PLANT-BASED DIET FOR MENTAL ABILITY

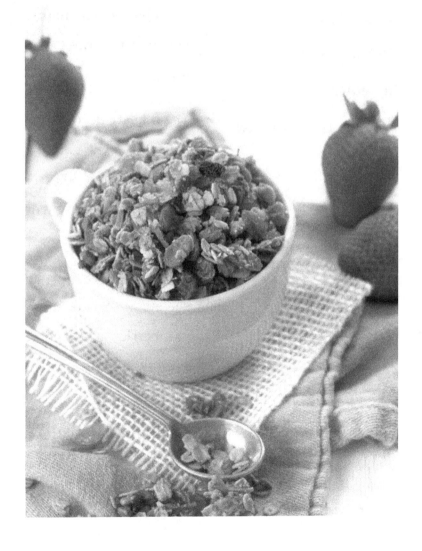

13.1 Green Goddess Granola

(Ready in about: 25 mins |Servings: 6 | Difficulty: Easy)

Ingredients:

- 1½ cups (135 g) rolled oats

- ¾ cup (120 g) buckwheat groats

- ¼ cup (35 g) pumpkin seeds

- ¼ cup (35 g) shelled hemp seeds

- ¼ cup (30 g) dried cranberries

- 2 tablespoons spirulina

- ¼ cup (3 or 4) Medjool dates,

- pitted and soaked in ½ cup (125 ml) water

- 4 tablespoons maple syrup raspberries.

Directions:

1. Preheat the oven to 150 ° C at a temperature of 300 ° F. Top a parchment bakery.

2. Mix oats, fruits, seeds of cotton, cranberries and pumpkin seeds.

3. In a large mixing cup, blend them together.

4. Remove the dates and put them in a

liquid, save four tablespoons soaking water.

5. Maple syrup processor and water reserved. Mix, so it's even.

6. In the bowl of mixture, powder it all.

7. Spread the mixture on the prepared baking sheet in a single layer, and stirring until gently and uniformly browned for about 20 minutes.

8. Remove from the oven, cool down and break into clusters.

9. Granola is stored for up to two weeks in an airtight container.

10. Serve with nice raspberries.

Nutritional Values:

- Calories (per serving) 280

- Protein 13.7 g

- Total fat 7.6 g

- Saturated fat 1.1 g

- carbohydrates 40.9 g

- dietary fibre 4.7 g

- sugars 13.6 g

- vitamins A

13.2 Green Smoothie Granola Bowls

(Ready in about: 7 mins | Servings: 2 | Difficulty: Easy)

Ingredients:

- 1 cup (70 g) kale,
- woody stems removed 1 cup (30 g) spinach
- 1 banana
- 1 cup (150 g) fresh or frozen mango chunks
- 1 tablespoon chia seeds
- 1 cup (250 ml) non-dairy milk (of choice)
- 1 cup (100 g) Green Goddess Granola
- 1 cup (125 g) fresh raspberries
- 2 tablespoons unsweetened coconut shreds
- 2 tablespoons goji berries.

Directions:

1. Cut the kale or split it into bits of morsel size. Kale, spinach, banana spot.

2. In a blender, combine mango, chia seeds and milk until creamy.

3. Split the smoothie into two bowls and squeeze 1/2 cup (50 g) each on top.

4. Divide between bowls and serve the raspberries, coconut shreds and goji berries.

Nutritional Values:

- Calories (per serving) 440

- protein 19.4 g

- Total fat 16.5 g

- saturated fat 9.2 g

- Carbohydrates 67 g

- dietary fibre 14.9 g

- sugars 38.1 g

CHAPTER 14. PLANT-BASED DIET FOR ENERGY BOOSTING

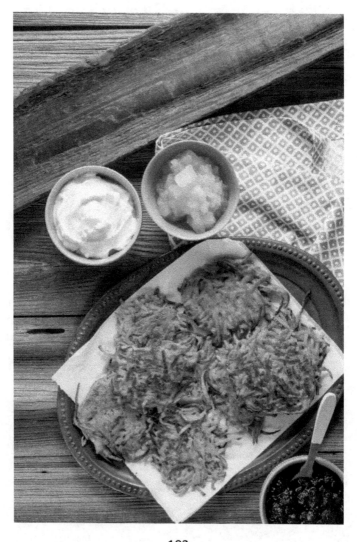

14.1 Sweet Potato Latkes

(Ready in about: 10 mins |Servings: 20 | Difficulty: Easy)

Ingredients:

- 1 large sweet potato, peeled and grated
- 2 tablespoons whole wheat flour
- 2 eggs, beaten
- 1/4 teaspoon garlic powder
- 1/4 teaspoon onion powder
- canola or vegetable oil, for pan searing
- apple sauce

Directions:

1. Place the first five Ingredients: into a dish and mix them completely.

2. Put on medium heat in a large sauté pot or griddle.

3. Heat 3–4 tbsp of oil in a jellyfish for 30 seconds or adequate to cover the bottom of the tank.

4. Cover the smooth potato mixture in a heaping table cubicle. Pat the mixture into a fine spherical patty with the back of a fork and shape (you don't

want them to be thick or they won't boil).

5. Five minutes cook or golden before they start to transform. Flip them over.

6. Continue cooking until the bottom is golden for another five minutes.

7. Drop the patties with a mixture of sweet potatoes onto a plate of paper towels and repeat them.

8. Serve and tasty patties.

* Cool off, mark and freeze then in the Ziploc bag. When ready, put it in an oven for 10 minutes at 300, or heat it in a dry pot until heated up or frosted in a refrigerator within 24 hours.

Nutritional Values:

- Calories 174.4

- Total Fat 9.5 g

- Saturated Fat 1.2 g

- Polyunsaturated Fat 2.5 g

- Monounsaturated Fat 5.0 g

- Cholesterol 93.4 mg

- Sodium 35.5 mg

- Potassium 176.2 mg

- Total Carbohydrate 18.5 g

- Dietary Fibre 2.6 g

- Sugars 0.0 g

- Protein 4.5 g

CHAPTER 15. WHOLE FOOD LUNCH AND DINNER RECIPES

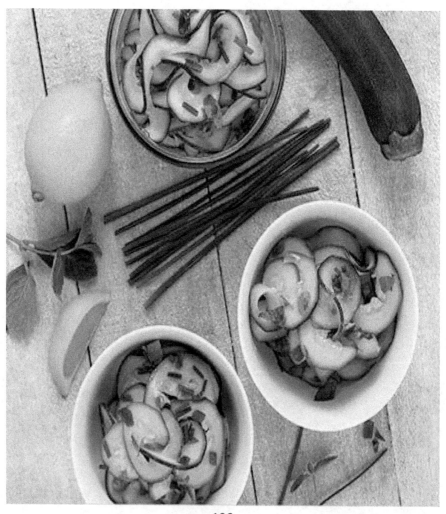

15.1 Courgette Ribbon Salad

(Ready in about: 20 mins |Servings: 4 | Difficulty: Easy)

Ingredients:

- juice 1 lemon

- 2 tbsp olive oil

- ½ small pack chives, chopped

- ½ small pack mint, chopped

- 300g courgettes

Directions:

1. Pour the citrus juice into a large bowl and season well with salt and pepper. Then apply the sliced herbs to the olive oil.

2. Place the courgette on its deep noodle connexion through the spiral and wear the ribbons in the dish. Put all together and serve straight away.

Nutritional Values:

- kcal 72

- fat 6g

- saturates 1g

- carbs 2g

- sugars 2g

- fibre 1g

- protein 2g

- salt 0g

15.4 Kale & Apple Soup with Walnuts

(Ready in about: 20 mins | Servings: 2 | Difficulty: Easy)

Ingredients:

- 8 walnut halves, broken into pieces
- 1 onion, finely chopped
- 2 carrots, coarsely grated
- 2 red apples, unpeeled and finely chopped
- 1 tbsp cider vinegar
- 500ml reduced-salt vegetable stock
- 200g kale, roughly chopped
- 20g pack of dried apple crisps

Directions:

1. Cook the noodles for 2-3 minutes in a dry, non-stick frying pan until they have become fried, regularly rotating to avoid their burning. Remove the heat and cool it.

2. Put in big cacao and bring to boil the onion, carrots, apples, vinegar and stock. Reduce the gas, stirring regularly and simmer for 10 minutes.

3. When the onion is transparent and the apples continue to

melt, apply the urine and fry for a further 2 minutes. Move carefully and mix very easily with a blender or liquidator. Place in bowls and serve with walnuts toasted and sprinkle with apple chips.

Nutritional Values:

- Calories kcal 403
- fat 21g
- saturates 2g
- carbs 36g
- sugars 25g
- fibre 9g
- protein 12g
- salt 0.8g

CHAPTER 16. DRINKS

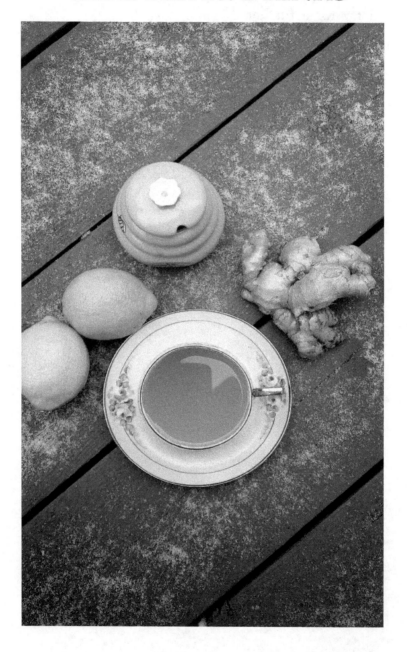

16.1 Honey Lemon Tea

(Ready in about: 3 mins |Servings: 1 | Difficulty: Easy)

Ingredients:

- 1 cup of water
- 2 teaspoons honey
- 1 teaspoon fresh lemon juice
- 1 teaspoon white sugar, or to taste

Directions:

1. Fill water into a cup. Add sugar and run 1 minute and 30 seconds in the microwave. Add the lemon juice and blend until the sweetness is dissolved, then add the sugar.

Nutritional Values:

- 62.9 Calories;
- Protein 0.1g;
- Carbohydrates 16.9g 6% Dv;
- Fat 0g;
- Cholesterol 0mg;
- Sodium 0.7mg.

16.2 Hong Kong Mango Drink

(Ready in about: 20 mins |Servings: 2 | Difficulty: Easy)

Ingredients:

- ½ cup small pearl tapioca

- 1 mango - peeled, seeded and diced
- 14 each's ice cubes
- ½ cup of coconut milk

Directions:

1. Cover a pot of water and bring high heat to a rolling boil. When the water heats, put in the pearls and go back to simmer. Cook exposed tapioca pearls, sometimes blending, for 10 minutes.

2. Copy and delete the heat for 30 minutes, allowing the perils to recover. Drain well in a lattice put in the drain, cover and cool.

3. In the mixer, place mango and ice and mix until it is creamy. Tape in 2 tall glasses the cooled tapioca pearls, then lay the mango over and add a 1/4 cup chocolate milk to each bottle.

Nutritional Values:

- 314.6 Calories;
- Protein 1.7g 4% Dv;
- Carbohydrates 52.9g 17% Dv;
- Fat 12.3g 19% Dv;
- Cholesterol 0mg;
- Sodium 14.2mg 1% Dv.

16.3 Hot Mocha Drink Mix

(Ready in about: 10 mins |Servings: 12 | Difficulty: Easy)

Ingredients:

- 2 tablespoons white sugar
- 2 tablespoons dry milk powder
- 2 tablespoons powdered non-dairy creamer
- 1 tablespoon unsweetened cocoa
- 2-1/4 teaspoons instant coffee granules

Directions:

1. Mix sugar, milk powder, cream, cacao and immediate coffee in a large cup. Until well combined, put together. Store in a jar that is sealed.

2. To be eaten, add 2 to 3 tablespoons of cocoa mixture to a taste of milk. Heat a cup of water per part.

Nutritional Values:

- 27.9 Calories;
- Protein 0.9g 2% Dv;
- Carbohydrates 5.2g 2% Dv;
- Fat 0.6g 1% Dv;
- Cholesterol 0.4mg;
- Sodium 12.5mg 1% Dv.

16.4 Honey Milk Tea - Hong Kong Style

(Ready in about: 15 mins |Servings: 1 | Difficulty: Easy)

Ingredients:

- 2 each's orange pekoe tea bags

- 1 cup boiling water

- 5 each's ice cubes

- 4 teaspoons sweetened condensed milk

- 3 teaspoons honey

Directions:

1. Soak the tea bags in hot water for about three to five minutes before the cooler turn's dark red. Throw the tea bags out and cool the tea.

2. In a bottle or cocktail shaker, mix ice cubes and condensed milk sweetened with honey. Bring the tea in and blend properly. A good and sweet dairy tea is ready for you to enjoy (if the tea still warms, the ice can melt; add more ice if desired.)

Nutritional Values:

- 150.6 Calories;

- Protein 2.1g 4% Dv;

- Carbohydrates 32.4g 11% Dv;

- Fat 2.2g 3% Dv;

- Cholesterol 8.7mg 3% Dv;

- Sodium 43.8mg 2% Dv.

CHAPTER 17. DESSERTS

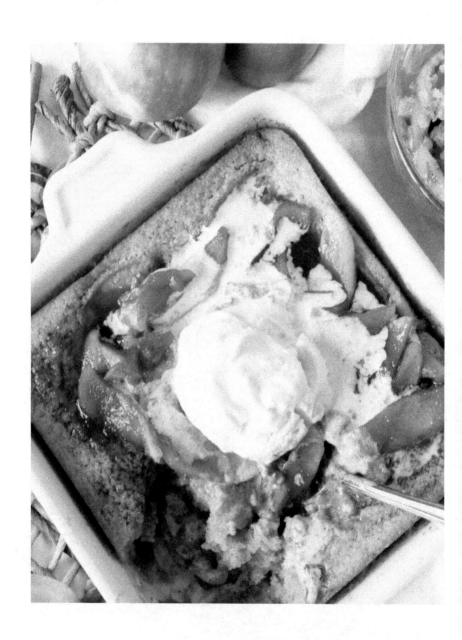

17.1 Virginia Apple Pudding

(Ready in about: 10 mins |Servings: 6 | Difficulty: Easy)

Ingredients:

- ½ cup butter, melted

- 1 cup white sugar

- 1 cup all-purpose flour

- 2 teaspoons baking powder

- ¼ teaspoon salt

- 1 cup milk

- 2 cups chopped, peeled apple

- 1 teaspoon ground cinnamon

Directions:

1. Oven pre-heats to 375 ° F (190 ° C). Oven pre-heat.

2. Pour butter, sugar, starch, pastry flour, salt and milk into a small baking dish until smooth.

3. Combine apples and cinnamon in a microwave-safe dish. Soft apples, 2 to 5 minutes, with a microwave. Pour apples into the batter's center.

4. Bake 30 minutes or until crispy in the pre-heated oven.

Nutritional Values:

- 384 calories;

- protein 3.8g 8% DV;

- carbohydrates 57.5g 19% DV;

- fat 16.4g 25% DV;

- cholesterol 43.9mg 15% DV;

- Sodium 343.3mg 14% DV.

17.2 Dessert Crepes

(Ready in about: 10 mins |Servings: 8 | Difficulty: Easy)

Ingredients

- 4 large eggs, lightly beaten

- 1 ⅓ cups milk

- 2 tablespoons butter, melted

- 1 cup all-purpose flour

- 2 tablespoons white sugar

- ½ teaspoon salt

Directions

1. Whisk together the eggs, milk, melted butter, sugar, and salt in a big bowl until smooth.

2. Over low cook, cook a medium-size skillet or crepe tray. With a brush or paper towel, grease the skillet with a small amount of butter or oil.

Spoon about 3 teaspoons of crepe batter into the hot pan using a serving spoon or small ladle, tilting the pan so that the bottom surface is uniformly coated. Cook on one side for 1 to 2 minutes, over medium heat, or until golden brown.
Immediately serve.

Nutritional values:

Per Serving:

- calories 164 ;

- protein 6.4g 13% DV;

- carbohydrates 17.2g 6% DV;

- fat 7.7g 12% DV;

- cholesterol 111.1mg 37% DV;

- sodium 234.5mg 9% DV.

Conclusion

Food is very important for human beings, however appreciation for a crucial concept has been lost; the nutrition. It is true that we live very hectic lifestyles where it is very common to find eating disorders and sleep disorders, not to mention other conditions such as diabetes or heart disease. It is then where we must lower our gaze and search our dishes for the answer.

Most of the diseases already mentioned are directly related to the type of diet of the person and by reading this cookbook, you manage to avoid diseases and you can develop more activities than you currently do. It is time to take charge of your diet and dare to discover preparations that will generate a notable change in your measurements and your health.

Remember that:

1.- It is never too late to start changing a habit.

2.- Vegetables do not have to be prepared in a boring way.

3.- You should have fun experimenting with your own recipes.

Start now and live the experience of having a healthier and simpler life!

CPSIA information can be obtained
at www.ICGtesting.com
Printed in the USA
LVHW020411120521
687183LV00009B/932